The Rise of Healthy Person

Secrets you never knew

By

Alam Mir

*To my beautiful Family, who gave me more
than I realized*

Acknowledgment

I would like to thank all of my friends, colleagues, trainers and specially team of Arfeen Khan who have contributed to this book.

I would especially like to thank Dr.Surinder Surya and Sh. Tiru Sameer of "Anyone Can Dance" fame.

Also, heartfelt thanks to our two enthusiastic children-Mohsin and Naushin for their contribution for designing cover of the book.

Contents

Chapter 5.5   How dance could be a major
                     contributory factor for mental
                     and physical health to rise as
                     healthy person

FOREWORD

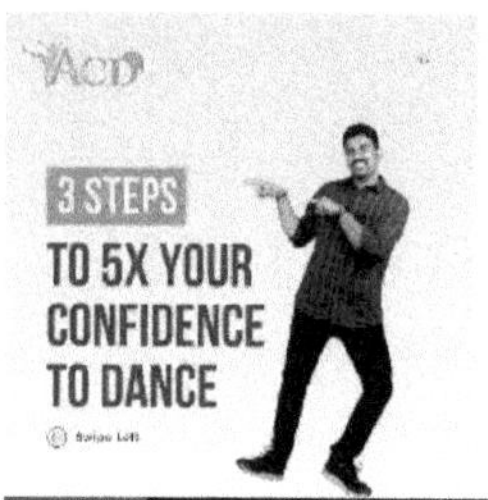

It is with immense pleasure that I pen this foreword for
"The Rise of Healthy Person" by Alam Mir. As someone
deeply invested in promoting wellness and dance through
my platform "Anyone Can Dance," I find this book a
profound and insightful guide to achieving holistic health.

Meeting Alam Mir, I was struck by his unwavering
commitment to health and wellness. His journey, as
chronicled in this book, is not just a personal testament
but a beacon for anyone aspiring to lead a healthier life.
The anecdotes and practical advice he offers resonate
deeply with my own experiences in the dance and fitness
world.

One of the most compelling aspects of Alam's narrative is his emphasis on a proactive approach to health. In our fast-paced world, where the tendency is to seek quick fixes, Alam's advocacy for natural and sustainable health practices is both refreshing and essential. His exploration of alternative methods to maintain and enhance health, beyond the realm of medication, aligns perfectly with my philosophy of using dance as a tool for mental and physical well-being.

This book is not just about health tips; it is a call to action. It encourages readers to take control of their health, embrace positive changes, and understand that true wellness comes from within. Alam's ability to interweave personal stories with practical advice makes this book a relatable and invaluable resource.

I am particularly moved by Alam's reflections on the importance of mindset and motivation in the pursuit of health. His insights on the power of visualization, affirmation, and the placebo effect are enlightening. These concepts are integral to my own practice as a dance trainer, where mental resilience and positive thinking are key components of my training programs.

"The Rise of Healthy Person" is more than just a book; it is a journey. It is an invitation to rise above the ordinary, to strive for a life of vitality and joy. Alam Mir has crafted a work that will inspire, educate, and motivate readers to transform their lives.

As you turn the pages of this remarkable book, I hope you find the same inspiration and determination that I did. May it guide you towards a healthier, happier, and more fulfilling life.

With warm regards,

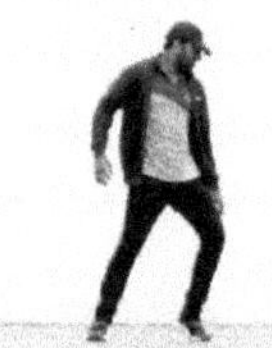

Tiru Sameer Yarlagadda
Chief Training Officer, Anyone Can Dance

The Rise of Healthy Person
-Secrets you never knew

A life without health is like a river without water.

PREFACE.......
A Memorable Reunion and the Journey to Health

It was a bright day in September 2016 when I found myself in our Gurgaon office, reunited with a colleague I hadn't seen in almost fifteen years. Meeting an old friend is always a delightful experience, filled with nostalgia and warmth. After a brief chat, we both returned to our daily routines.

The following Sunday, he invited me to his home in Dwarka for lunch. Meeting his family and wife after so many years was a surreal experience. Her initial reaction was one of pleasant surprise, "Alam da looks just the same as he did 15 years ago."

We enjoyed a sumptuous lunch, featuring a special Bengali dish called macher jhol (fish curry). Later, we visited another colleague in the Dwarka area. His wife echoed the same sentiment, "Alam, you look just the same as we saw you 17 years ago." Two women, two identical compliments!

At 54, maintaining the same appearance after so many years sparked questions within me. Is this a sign of good health? Is there something about my lifestyle that acts as an antidote to aging? I've always been conscious about health, often sharing fitness tips with others. These compliments made me ponder the results of my efforts.

The book you're holding unfolds some fascinating real-life experiences. Before we delve deeper, let me share what my inner voice says. As the world grapples with the COVID-19 pandemic, it has become clear that a robust immune system is essential. We must focus on personal health to rise to the next level of wellness.

While destiny remains unpredictable, we can take control of our health proactively, rather than relying solely on medication. Through this book, I hope to contribute to the community, offering insights to help you maintain good health.

During a 50-hour marathon NLP Master Practitioner training course, the trainer was astonished by my age. He publicly suggested that I serve as a meta-model for fitness and health. One participant even remarked that I resembled James

Bond in real life! What a compliment! Later on, with a firm belief on self, with visulaisation and affirmation that I could run half marathon in Guwahati, I recently completed 21 KM Half marathon also at my late fifties.

This book aims to guide you on your journey to becoming a healthier person. Let's turn the pages and discover how you too can rise to the next level of health and wellness.

DISCLAIMER

The ideas, concepts, and opinions expressed in this book are intended to be used for educational purposes only. This book sold with the understanding that the author and publisher are not rendering medical advice of any kind, nor is this book intended to replace medical advice, nor to diagnose, prescribe or treat any disease, condition, illness, or injury.

It is imperative that before beginning any diet or exercise program, including any aspect of *The Rise of Healthy Person*, you should receive full medical clearance from a licensed physician. Author and publisher claim no responsibility to any person or entity for any liability, loss, or damage caused or alleged to be caused directly or indirectly as a result of the use, application, or interpretation of the material in this book.

Introduction

"Happiness is the highest form of health."
— Dalai Lama

Anti-Aging: Is It Possible to Turn Back the Clock?

You may have noticed that many Bollywood actors and actresses, well past their seventies, continue to thrive both in movies and society. Consider these legends:

- **Dilip Kumar (DOB: December 11, 1922) – 95 Years**
- **Chandrashekhar (DOB: July 07, 1923) – 94 Years**
- **Kamini Kaushal (DOB: January 16, 1927) – 91 Years**
- **Ramesh Deo (DOB: January 30, 1929) – 89 Years**
- **Gulzar (DOB: August 18, 1929) – 88 Years**
- **Lata Mangeshkar (DOB: September 28, 1929) – 88 Years**
- **Asha Bhosle (DOB: September 8, 1933) – 84 Years**
- **Prem Chopra (DOB: September 23, 1935) – 82 Years**
- **Dharmendra (DOB: December 8, 1935) – 82 Years**
- **Jeetendra (DOB: April 7, 1942) – 76 Years**
- **Amitabh Bachchan (DOB: October 11, 1942) – 75 Years**

These stars still dominate the celebrity world, defying age with their enduring vitality.

Globally, as of June 10, 2020, the oldest known living

person is Kane Tanaka of Japan, aged 117 years and

160 days. The oldest living man is Dumitru Comănescu of Romania, aged 111 years and 215 days. Jeanne Calment of France holds the record for the longest-lived person, passing away at 122 years and 164 days in 1997. Calment humorously remarked that God must have forgotten about her.

How is such longevity possible? Anti-aging has become a buzzword, with many seeking ways to extend life and improve health. Before diving into the latest breakthroughs in anti-aging, let's first understand aging itself.

What is Aging?

Aging is often apparent through changes in appearance — grey hair, wrinkled skin, and other visible signs. These reflect underlying physiological changes, such as decreased pigment production in hair follicles and reduced skin elasticity. While cosmetic surgery can alter appearance, it doesn't change the underlying physiology.

For women, aging is often associated with decreased fertility, culminating in menopause. This is why women may be sensitive about their age, preferring to avoid reminders of this inevitable process. Aging also weakens bones and muscles, increasing the risk of fractures and reducing physical strength.

On a cellular level, aging reduces the body's response to hormones. High insulin or thyroid hormone levels, for example, are less effective if cells no longer respond properly. Mitochondria, the "powerhouses" of cells, become less efficient, leading to higher rates of illness and disease. Aging exponentially increases the risk of disease and death, with conditions like heart attacks becoming more common in the elderly.

Aging itself is not a disease, but it increases the likelihood of developing diseases, making it a prime target for interventions. Chronological age is irreversible, but physiological age can be influenced by various factors. Aging is essentially the accumulation of damage, and while young bodies repair this damage effectively, this ability diminishes with age.

The good news is that researchers in Japan have found that human aging might be delayed or even reversed at the cellular level. Anti-aging drugs are in development, but why wait for them when we can create our own anti-aging solutions through lifestyle and nutrition?

We don't have to wait for expensive, potentially inaccessible drugs. We have the tools within us to combat aging. The challenge is to address our current health conditions and take proactive steps towards long-term vitality.

The Challenges of Health and Marriage

After the whirlwind of a dramatic wedding, everything seemed to be going well. We were happy, both working, raising kids, and living life much like any other married couple. But after ten years of marriage, my wife began showing some concerning health symptoms: hunger and fatigue, slow-healing wounds, and weight loss. Recognizing these as potential signs of diabetes, we decided to get her tested.

The diagnosis was clear: Type 2 diabetes. Additionally, her frequent mood swings and high blood pressure compounded our concerns. The real struggle began with her reaction: "Why me?" she asked, angry and frustrated. The burden of her frustration often fell on me, the nearest available target.

In relationships, it's often wise to remain silent in the face of certain "why's." So, I kept quiet, knowing that illness is a complex topic with many variables — everyone's body, mind, upbringing, and family history are different. The challenge we faced was accepting and acknowledging the diagnosis. My wife was not ready to accept her condition, repeatedly asking, "Why me? Why do I have to suffer?"

She voiced her frustration, noting how she bore the brunt of running the household, her job, and taking care of the kids, while I, in her eyes, seemed relaxed. The responsibilities and stress of our dual-income household undoubtedly added to her anxiety and health issues.

To help her understand and accept her condition, I delved into research. Diabetes and high blood pressure are among the most common diseases in India. One in six people with diabetes worldwide is from India, making our country second only to China in the number of diabetics. By 2025, three-quarters of the world's 300 million adults with diabetes will be in non-industrialized countries, with India and China alone accounting for nearly a third.

Explaining these statistics provided some relief. She realized she was not alone. Type 2 diabetes, I explained, often results from a combination of genetic and environmental factors. Asian Indians, in particular, have a higher degree of insulin resistance compared to Caucasians. Socio-economic development has led to lifestyle changes, including physical inactivity, poor diets, and high levels of mental stress, all contributing to diabetes.

Physical inactivity and obesity are significant risk factors for diabetes, especially in urban areas. Studies show that overweight and central obesity are strongly linked to diabetes, even among children. High intake of saturated fats also increases the risk of developing diabetes.

Despite understanding more about diabetes, my wife's "why" regarding her high blood pressure persisted. Hypertension is a major health issue in modern-day living, with one in four adults in India affected. This condition, often silent in its early stages, is a leading risk factor for cardiovascular disease. Routine checks usually reveal its presence, earning it the moniker "silent killer" due to its hidden impact on vital organs like the kidneys, heart, and brain.

One in five young adults in India has high blood pressure. This equates to around 80 million people—more than the entire UK population. Hypertension is defined as systolic blood pressure (BP) ≥140 mmHg or diastolic BP ≥90 mmHg, or being on treatment for hypertension.

After learning about the prevalence of these conditions, my wife felt a bit more secure knowing that she was not alone. Many people, including men, suffer from diabetes and high blood pressure. This shared understanding brought some comfort as we navigated this challenging phase together.

Chapter 1.1   Wife is diagnosed with Type B diabetes and high Blood pressure.

Doctors won't make you healthy. Nutritionists won't make you slim. Teachers won't make you smart. Gurus won't make you calm. Mentors won't make you rich. Trainers won't make you fit. Ultimately, you have to take responsibility. Save yourself.

Naval Ravikant

After high voltage dramatic marriage, everything was going fine. We are happy. Both working. Having kids and running our life just like any other married couples.

But after ten years of marriage, the wife started showing some health symptoms. Like Hunger and fatigue. wounds that are slow to heal, weight loss.

As all these symptoms are the sign of diabetes, we thought it's better to get the laboratory tests done.

So we did.

And, Result declared its Type 2 diabetes.

As the wife is having frequent mood change and hypertension, her blood pressure also shows she is having high blood pressure.

Problem started.

Her first reaction was, why? why me?

The second problem, out of anger and frustration, the reaction of the problem will divert to only available person.

That is me.

Yes, in such a situation, the only person you can make the victim of anything.

That is the husband!

Why I have to suffer, why not you?

No answer from me.

As you know, in a relationship, it's better to keep quiet for many "why's.

I also kept quiet.

Because it's a subject of much research.

Who will fall ill and who not, no one can tell.

Also, everyone's body and mind condition and also upbringing and also, family history was different.

The problem, we faced at that time was to accepting and acknowledging.

The wife was not at all ready to accept it. She is not acknowledging that she had these diseases Diabetes and High blood pressure.

Why me?

Why in this world, only I had to suffer?

 Why not you.

As I had to take all tension of running home, my work, taking care of kids and whatnot.

So, all responsibilities and tension, anxiety, and worry I was taking and so I had to suffer. You all husbands are relaxed.

Now, things come out not singular. It is in plural forms.

No tension. So, why you have to suffer.

I had to listen.

And, causes are genuine too. Because, when both husband and wife are working. It is so true that the wife has to take extra responsibilities in addition to her office works. That is her first home!

So, there is every possibility of developing extra anxiety and stress bombs. Some can manage well and cope up with the situation and some cannot.

Result?

Multiple.

But, why diabetes and high pressure.

I had to study a lot just to make my wife convinced to accept and acknowledge that diabetes and high blood pressure are now the most common diseases in India. Even, globally.

Other than asking why, if we go a bit deeper, then only, we can feel contented and move forward to the next course of action.

So, our quest begins with diabetes and high blood pressure.

Data is shocking.

One in six people with diabetes worldwide is from India. This positions India among the top ten countries for diabetes, ranking second with an estimated 77 million diabetics. China tops the list with over 116 million diabetics.

Diabetes, a global public health problem, is now emerging as a pandemic and by the year 2025, three-quarters of the world's 300 million adults with diabetes will be in non-industrialized countries and almost a third in India and China alone.

When data were described in detail to the wife, she got a bit of relief.

With a big sigh, her body posture said: I am not the only one!

Reasons?

One of the important factors contributing to increased Type 2 diabetes in Asian Indians is the fact that they have a greater degree of insulin resistance compared to Caucasians.

The epidemic increase in diabetes in India along with various studies on migrant and native Indians indicate that Indians have an increased predilection to diabetes which could well be due to a greater genetic predisposition to diabetes in Indians. Genetic susceptibility appears to play an important role in the occurrence of Type 2 diabetes.

However, Type 2 diabetes is known to be a multifactorial disease caused by a complex interplay of genetic (inheritance) and environmental (diet and lifestyle) factors that influence many intermediate traits of relevance to the diabetic phenotype.

Socio-economic development has resulted in a dramatic change in lifestyle from traditional to modern, leading to physical inactivity due to technological advancement, affluence leading to consumption of diets rich in fat, sugar and calories and a high level of mental stress.

I had to emphasise the word "Mental stress" while describing the above research on diabetes to my wife!

All these could adversely influence insulin sensitivity and lead to obesity. Some called diabetes a Rich Person's disease.

There is ample epidemiological evidence to demonstrate that physical inactivity as an independent risk factor is fuelling the epidemic of Type 2 diabetes, predominantly in the urban areas. Another study showed that overweight/obesity and central obesity were significantly associated with diabetes. Obesity has been on the increase in children, which might play a causative role in the escalating prevalence of diabetes in the young.

This increased occurrence of overweight in childhood may be the first sign of insulin resistance and future metabolic syndrome.

A high intake of saturated fatty acids has been associated with an increased risk of developing impaired glucose tolerance (IGT) and diabetes and of progression to diabetes from IGT, whereas unsaturated fatty acids, especially n-3 polyunsaturated fatty acids, have been inversely associated with the risk of diabetes.

Though my wife seemed a bit relaxed her "why" to suffer from High blood pressure haunted me.

Why??

Being husband, you have to answer back all "why", otherwise.......

After studying about High blood pressure, I tried to make my wife convinced that you are not alone.

Hypertension (High Blood Pressure) is among the major scourges of modern-day living. According to WHO estimates, the prevalence of Hypertension in India is about 25 per cent, i.e., one in four adults in India suffer from hypertension. This high prevalence coupled with inadequate knowledge about the disease makes it a guaranteed recipe for disaster.

Hypertension is the most important risk factor for cardiovascular morbidity and mortality. There is limited data on hypertension prevalence in India.

As you may be knowing, Blood is the oxygen and nutrient-carrying vehicle in the human body. To reach its point of utilization it needs to be pumped by the human heart. This mechanical activity of the heart produces a pressure which is called *Blood Pressure*. It is measured in *millimetres of mercury.*

A national-level survey was conducted with fixed one-day blood pressure measurement camps across 24 states and union territories of India. One in five young adults in India has high blood pressure, according to research presented at the 70th Annual Conference of the Cardiological Society of India (CSI). That equates to around 80 million people, which is more than the entire UK population.

 Hypertension was defined as systolic blood pressure (BP) ≥140 mmHg or a diastolic BP ≥90 mmHg or on treatment for hypertension.

Hypertension often does not produce any discomfort or illness for a patient in the early phase of the illness. It usually remains 'silent' and is detected only when after a routine check-up. The reason why it is called a "silent killer" is that even though the individual does not have any complaints, hypertension keeps affecting the vital organs such as kidneys, heart and brain. The first manifestation of hypertension may be heart or kidney failure or a debilitating paralytic stroke.

Is not its shocking news: 1 in every 5 Indians affected by Hypertension!!

Given the current situation in our country, one comforting thought for my wife is that she isn't alone in her struggle with diabetes and high blood pressure; there are other men, aside from her husband, facing the same health issues

Chapter 1.2 Not accepting and acknowledging the diseases for 6 months to start medication

The most dangerous thing, when you have a serious mental illness, is convincing yourself that you don't have it. And you see it all the time. People get on medication, and they feel better, and they stop taking it. And some flirt with unreality on some levels. But it feels so convincing to them that it feels real.

Noah Hawley

The diagnosis of diabetes and high blood pressure was not the real problem. The problem arose when my wife vowed not to take any medication, insisting she could cure herself through natural remedies alone. I had to admire her strong willpower, but I knew that managing these conditions without medication would be challenging, especially given her lifestyle.

As a working woman and housewife, my wife's life was filled with tension and anxiety — two major contributors to diabetes and high blood pressure. Research shows these are lifestyle diseases, and without a lifestyle change, improvement is unlikely. But was it possible for her to change her lifestyle given her responsibilities? Not at all. Without medication, her symptoms could worsen.

Denial, in this context, is a way of protecting oneself from painful truths. Initially, it can provide time to adjust to stressful situations, but it has a dark side. Denial can prevent acknowledging a problem, facing facts, and understanding the consequences. This coping mechanism can delay taking necessary action, leading to serious long-term consequences.

When you're in denial, you:

- Won't acknowledge a difficult situation
- Avoid facing the facts of a problem
- Downplay the possible consequences

Short-term denial can be helpful, allowing the mind to absorb distressing information gradually. However, prolonged denial prevents taking appropriate action, such as seeking medical treatment. This can lead to untreated conditions worsening over time.

Understanding human psychology, I advised my wife during her denial phase to:

- Honestly examine what she fears

- Consider the potential negative consequences of not taking action
- Express her fears and emotions
- Identify irrational beliefs about her situation
- Journal about her experience
- Open up to a trusted friend or loved one
- Participate in a support or mastermind group

It can be frustrating when someone you love is in denial about a serious issue like not taking medication for diabetes and high blood pressure. I knew it would take time for her to face the facts, so I took a step back while letting her know I was open to discussing the subject. This approach might eventually give her the security to move forward.

If a loved one is in denial about a serious health issue, forcefully bringing up the issue might be difficult and could lead to confrontations. Instead, listen and offer support without trying to force treatment. This gentle approach can provide the necessary support for them to acknowledge and address their condition.

Chapter 1.3 Why the only wife to suffer from these common diseases why not the husband

Your health is what you make of it. Everything you do and think either adds to the vitality, energy and spirit you possess or takes away from it.

Anonymous

When my wife questioned why she was the one suffering from diabetes and high blood pressure, while her husband seemed unaffected, there was no simple answer. Such questions prompt a deeper exploration into the underlying issues to find solutions. When you deeply love and care for someone, leaving no stone unturned in search of answers is instinctual.

It's common for people to initially struggle with accepting a new diagnosis. This discomfort is natural, and most eventually come to terms with their condition. However, in some cases, rejection persists long-term, driven not by denial but by a condition known as anosognosia — a term meaning "lack of awareness or insight" in Greek.

Anosognosia goes beyond simple denial or stubbornness; it reflects a neurological inability to perceive one's own medical reality despite clear evidence and professional diagnosis. This condition is often associated with changes in the brain, particularly affecting the frontal lobe responsible for self-image and perception.

Over time, conditions like schizophrenia or bipolar disorder can lead to remodelling of frontal lobe tissue, impairing the ability to update one's self-perception and acknowledge new medical information. This cognitive barrier can be frustrating for both the individual and their loved ones, who may struggle to understand why the person doesn't take their condition seriously.

A hallmark of anosognosia is a persistent lack of awareness or acceptance of one's medical condition, even in the face of overwhelming evidence. Distinguishing between anosognosia and other responses like denial requires careful observation of behaviours over time, noting variations in insight that may fluctuate.

Navigating such complexities often leads to seeking medical advice and consultations to better understand and address the underlying issues. Seeking professional guidance becomes essential in managing conditions where awareness and acceptance pose significant challenges.

In conclusion, understanding and compassion are crucial in supporting individuals grappling with their health conditions, whether facing denial, anosognosia, or other responses. By acknowledging these complexities, we can approach diagnosis and treatment with empathy and clarity, ensuring effective support and care.

Chapter 1.4 Is ultimately medication the only way to get cured?

Bad things do happen; how I respond to them defines my character and the quality of my life. I can choose to sit in perpetual sadness, immobilized by the gravity of my loss, or I can choose to rise from the pain and treasure the most precious gift I have - life itself.

Walter Anderson

For nearly six months, my wife wrestled with a crucial decision: whether to begin medication for her newly diagnosed diabetes and high blood pressure. Despite showing clear symptoms like mood swings and heightened stress, she hesitated. Her reluctance stemmed from a fear that once she started medication, there would be no turning back—an irreversible commitment echoing through her researched knowledge of these conditions worldwide.

Navigating this dilemma called for emotional validation—a process I began to apply, drawing on my understanding of its impact. Emotional validation isn't about agreeing with someone's emotions but acknowledging and accepting them without dismissal. This approach was pivotal as my wife grappled with questions like "Why me, why not my husband?" Slowly, the concept of emotional validation started to resonate with her, highlighting its significant role in our journey.

Emotional validation communicates acceptance, strengthens relationships, and aids in better emotional regulation. By validating her emotions, I showed that her feelings were understood and respected, fostering a sense of support during her struggle. Validating statements like "I can see how you would feel that way" or "I'm here for you" became crucial in affirming her experience without judgment.

Applying emotional validation required careful consideration of body language, empathy, and thoughtful questioning. It was essential to create an open and supportive environment, free from blame or defensiveness. Despite these efforts, the turning point came after consulting local doctors, who outlined potential complications if her conditions remained untreated.

The gravity of potential complications, including ketoacidosis and long-term organ damage, painted a stark reality. Learning that India bears the title of the diabetes capital of the world further underscored the urgency for treatment. The doctor's account of a stroke due to missed high blood pressure medication left no room for doubt— medication was imperative.

With these revelations, the decision was made, and medication began. It marked a pivotal moment in our journey—a testament to the power of understanding, acceptance, and informed action in facing health challenges head-on. Through emotional validation and informed medical guidance, we embarked on a path toward managing and improving my wife's health, navigating challenges with resilience and hope.

Chapter 2.1 Once dependant on medication, why it's difficult to overcome dependency

I do believe in the old saying, 'What does not kill you makes you stronger.' Our experiences, good and bad, make us who we are. By overcoming difficulties, we gain strength and maturity.

Angelina Jolie

After 14 years of taking medication for diabetes and high blood pressure, my wife's condition seemed stable. But the side effects of these medications? Can anyone deny them? Absolutely not. They're always there, lurking in the background, causing who knows what internal complications.

Fed up, I told my wife to stop taking the medicine. Her reaction? "Do you want me to die? These are my lifeline! I can't stop. I have to take them for the rest of my life. There's no other way."

Why is it so hard to stop once it's ingrained in our body and mind? Over time, people can become dependent on these medications. It's almost like an addiction. Quitting feels impossible because the drugs change how our brains work.

Medications, like those for diabetes and high blood pressure, travel through our bloodstream to the brain, altering how messages are sent. They play with our neurotransmitters – the brain's communication chemicals. Some meds boost dopamine, the pleasure chemical, making us feel good and want more. But when dopamine levels drop, we feel flat and depressed.

Repeated dopamine depletion can damage the brain's pathways, especially those in the prefrontal cortex, which help us think and make decisions. This makes medication use almost automatic, and stopping feels unbearable.

I know it's hard to quit, but you don't have to do it alone. Our brains adapt to the changes these drugs bring, making it difficult to give them up. Like my wife, many people struggle to break free from this dependence.

To change things up, I suggested to my wife that we stop checking her sugar levels and blood pressure every month. I shared my story of recovering from an umbilical hernia without surgery or extra medicine. Sometimes, you have to reach a point where you say, "Enough is enough!"

Chapter 2.2   Inspiration from my own experience of   repairing an umbilical hernia without surgery.

Helping those who have been struck by unforeseeable misfortunes is fundamentally different from making dependency a way of life.

Thomas Sowell

Every day, in every way, I'm getting better and better. Say it with me: Every day, in every way, I'm getting better and better.

You might be surprised to know that in the 18th century, French psychologist and pharmacist Emile Coue used this very phrase to treat thousands of patients with different diseases — and his success rate was astounding!

Coue believed that most mental and physical illnesses stemmed from a person's thinking. So, when we repeat positive affirmations, real changes happen in our bodies. Why? Because words have incredible power.

Believe it or not, words can shape our reality. Emile Coue knew this well, and that's why he had such profound success treating patients. If only we could use these century-old techniques today for healing!

But it's not too late, my friends. We have the freedom to use whatever techniques work for us, naturally curing ourselves instead of relying on medicines with side effects.

Let's demonstrate the power of words together. Just say, "Yes!" The most positive word there is. Can you feel the surge of positive energy? Let's do it again. "Yes!"

But remember, you have to say it congruently. What does that mean? It means saying it with your whole being—your posture, gesture, and emotion should all align with your words.

Now, with these positive words and a feeling of confidence, power, and energy, let's say "YES" again and feel the difference inside us. Does it empower your state of being? I'm sure it does because I'm living proof.

After two years in Algeria, a full-body check-up in Delhi revealed a 10 mm gall bladder stone. I was sceptical about surgery, having successfully treated ailments naturally. But the doctor explained that the stone's location made natural treatment impossible, so I had the surgery.

Everything seemed fine until a week later when I developed infections in my belly incisions. The doctor prescribed medication and frequent visits for treatment, but the infection worsened. The doctor suspected TB, and I began TB medication, only to suffer severe side effects.

Eventually, a visit to Apollo Chennai revealed the infection was spreading internally, requiring another surgery. After three months of antibiotics, a lump formed at my umbilical area—a hernia. The doctor recommended another surgery.

That was when I remembered Emile Coue's quote: Every day, in every way, I'm getting better and better. If Coue treated patients with this phrase because words had power, why not try it myself?

I came across Masaru Emoto's water experiments, which showed that positive words could change the physical structure of water. Our bodies are over 70%

water, so positive words can have a profound effect on us.

I reframed Coue's quote to: Every day, in every way, my umbilical hernia is getting reduced and reduced. I repeated this affirmation every morning and evening, visualizing my hernia shrinking.

Consistently, day after day, month after month, year after year, I did this. After five years, my umbilical hernia is almost constricted. Manageable. That's the power of words!

Chapter 2.3   Is there another method to look well besides taking medication?

I'm learning not to hold on so tightly to my solitude. It's not an economical way to work. A driver would call it 'white-knuckling.' If you're holding on to the wheel so tightly, it's going to lock up you're driving. Releasing myself from trying to control everything has been part of growing up.

Ben Foster

Seeing myself heal from a probable third surgery for an umbilical hernia inspired my wife to take a new approach to her diabetes and high blood pressure. She realized that taking medicines for these conditions has no end. She began studying alternative ways to treat her ailments.

Alternative medicine systems share the belief that the body can heal itself, often using techniques that involve the mind, body, and spirit. CAM (Complementary and Alternative Medicine) practices include alternative medical systems, mind-body interventions, biologically-based treatments, manipulative methods, and energy therapies.

As part of her new approach, my wife stopped checking her sugar and blood pressure levels every month. This helped change her mindset. Constantly seeing those reports made her believe she had a problem. The solution? Break the pattern—stop seeing the reports!

With her roots in Majuli, the world's largest river island in Assam, she researched the island's medicinal plants. A study by P. Hazarika, B.K. Pandey, and Y.C. Tripathi documented antidiabetic herbs from Majuli, revealing fascinating findings about plants used to treat diabetes and high blood pressure.

In many developing countries, herbal treatments are culturally accepted and economically viable. The World Health Organization lists 20,000 medicinal plants used worldwide. The Majuli study documented indigenous knowledge of plants with hypoglycaemic activities, providing clues for isolating bioactive compounds for clinical trials.

Thirty medicine men and diabetic patients,
including three women, were interviewed about
their use of local plants for diabetes treatment.
From 2003 to 2007, the research team gathered

information by interviewing elderly individuals, local herbal doctors, and household women in Majuli.

Here are some of the plants documented:

1. **Adhatoda vasica Nees (Tita bhak)**: Extract from fresh leaves mixed with water, used thrice daily for one month to lower blood glucose levels.

2. **Azadirachta indica L. (Maha neem)**: Aqueous leaf extract or powdered leaves, sometimes five fresh leaves taken on an empty stomach in the morning.

3. **Catharanthus roseus (Nayantara)**: Ground extract from flowers and leaves, taken in small teaspoons.

4. **Emblica officinalis Gaertn. (Amlokhi)**: Juice from mature fruits with honey, taken twice daily.

5. **Enhydra fluctuans Lour. (Haleshi sak)**: Leafy vegetable used as a decoction for controlling blood sugar.

6. **Heliotropium indicum (Hatisuria bon)**: Aerial parts used by Deori communities for diabetes.

7. **Zingiber officinale Rosc. (Ada/Zinger)**: Warm water extract of ginger rhizome, used regularly to control sugar levels.

Fascinated by these medicinal plants, my wife planted Nayantara plant at home and used it as described. Now, her diabetes and high blood pressure are completely under control.

Chapter 2.4   What drives us all the time to get demotivated in respect of health issues

When humor can be made to alternate with melancholy, one has a success, but when the same things are funny and melancholic at the same time, it's just wonderful.

Francois Truffaut

Feeling demotivated can be one of the worst feelings in the world. You feel lost, without direction, and lacking the drive to change your situation. If you're reading this, you might be wondering why you're experiencing this and what you can do to overcome it.

Here are 10 reasons why you might be feeling demotivated:

1. **You Are Working Without Purpose** The biggest reason for demotivation is living without goals or intent. Without a clear purpose, you may feel like you're just going through the motions. The good news is, this can be fixed. Figure out what you want from life and set specific, achievable goals. I found my purpose after seeing my father

bedridden before he passed away. I vowed to stay fit and independent. What about you?

2. **Your Lack of Motivation Stems from Fear** Fear of progress can keep you stuck, leading to discontent and demotivation. Whether in your personal or professional life, this fear creates obstacles that become harder to overcome with time.

3. **You're Doing Things for the Wrong Reasons** Your body can sense when you're not aligned with your actions. Ask yourself if you're doing things for the right reasons.

4. **You Take on Too Much and Are Overwhelmed** Ambition is great, but taking on too much can lead to burnout. It's important to pace yourself and take things slowly and steadily.

5. **You May Be Dealing with Symptoms of a Mental Illness** Mental illness can sometimes go unnoticed. My wife, for example, stopped taking her diabetes medication for six months, which affected her motivation.

6. **Your Goals Are Too Big** Having goals is crucial, but they need to be realistic. I once

aimed to have a body like Salman Khan but realized it was too ambitious.

7. **You're Engaging in Self-Sabotage** If you believe you lack the skills to improve or think others doubt you, you might sabotage your own efforts. This can stunt your growth and prevent you from achieving your potential.

8. **You Feel You Should Have Accomplished More by Now** Many people pressure themselves to have achieved more. Instead of dwelling on the past, focus on the future. After recovering from my umbilical hernia, I now aim to stay fit and inspire others.

9. **You Have a Habit of NOT Doing Anything** Some people simply choose not to act on their potential. This habit leads to demotivation and difficulty in getting things done.

10. **You're Settling and Refusing to Push Your Limits** Settling for less can also cause demotivation. Instead, push your limits and strive for what you're capable of achieving.

Act as If You Feel Motivated

You can trick yourself into feeling motivated by changing your behavior. Every morning, I follow Hal Elrod's six-morning miracle habits, known as SAVERS:

- **S for Silence**: Start with morning prayer or meditation. I ask my daughter, Naushin, to focus on the birds chirping outside.
- **A for Affirmation**: Say positive things to yourself. I encourage Naushin to affirm, "I am the best, I am the most intelligent girl, today will be the best day," and the magic phrase, "Every day in every way, I am getting better and better."
- **V for Visualization**: Create a positive mental picture. I ask Naushin to visualize doing excellently in her upcoming tests.
- **E for Exercise**: A bit of morning exercise goes a long way, and Naushin never skips it.
- **R for Reading**: Make reading a habit. Naushin reads every morning from Vijay Agarwal's book, "The Hanuman Who Never Fails."

- **S for Scribing**: Write something about yourself. Naushin keeps a journal of the previous day's events.

By consistently practicing these SAVERS habits, you can achieve extraordinary results, just like Hal Elrod!

Chapter 3.1 You will be inspired to feel strongly about staying in shape by Dr. Surinder Surya's narrative.

It is health that is real wealth and not pieces of gold and silver.

<u>*Mahatma Gandhi*</u>

You ask any health expert, and they will tell you that to maintain or improve your health, aim for 150 minutes per week—or at least 30 minutes on all or most days of the week—of moderate physical activity. Moderate activities are ones that you can talk—but not sing—while doing, such as brisk walking or dancing. These activities speed up your heart rate and breathing.

But do you think exercise alone is sufficient?

To delve deeper into the secret of maintaining health, I found none other than Dr. Surinder Surya from our Incredible You Mastermind group, who, at 58, maintains excellent health. Dr. Surinder Surya, an MBBS doctor with a fellowship in aesthetic medicine, is a soft-spoken general practitioner with over 25 years of experience. He is also the District General Secretary of IMA, State Joint Secretary of

IMA, and President of the Sonologist Association of Himachal Pradesh.

At 58, Dr. Surya not only feels like he's 35 but looks like too!

When asked about his health and fitness regimen, Dr. Surya shared his story. At 16, he suffered from a persistent runny nose, always carrying tablets in his pocket. One day, he watched a Russian TV program where a mind power expert bent a spoon with mental focus. Inspired, Dr. Surya began visualizing and affirming that his runny nose would be cured. After two years, it was gone!

Since then, Dr. Surya has consistently practiced positive affirmations, saying, "I am fit. I am positive."

Later, he developed hypothyroidism, a condition where the thyroid doesn't produce enough hormones, leading to weight gain and fatigue. Despite this, Dr. Surya has maintained his weight at around 67-68 kg for the last 20 years. He takes one tablet daily and practices written affirmations morning and evening:

- I am fit physically.

- I am fit mentally.
- I am fit psychologically.
- I am fit spiritually.
- I am fit autonomically.
- I am fit hormonally.
- I am 35 years old.

When asked about his secret, Dr. Surya beautifully described his mantra for living healthy: "My positivity is my biggest secret. I kept telling myself and feeding my subconscious mind that I am 35 years old. For the last 22 years, I have looked and felt 35. If you meet me, you'd think I am 35. My subconscious mind kept me the way I wanted. This is why I am healthy, fit, and youthful. This is my mantra!"

As Dr. Surya explains, our subconscious mind is much stronger than our conscious mind. By affirming with deep feeling, we can influence our bodies. Even at 58, he doesn't look his age!

This is the secret of his health and fitness. If a well-established doctor can stay fit through positive affirmations, why can't we?

Chapter 3.2   You have the right to feel healthy.

If we can soften our hearts, and if we can access the pure and simple aspect of our nature, then we can regain the realization that everything we need is already inside us and anything is attainable.

Yehuda Berg

As we are born into this world, we have every right to feel healthy and grow as healthy individuals. It's our birthright. No one can take that away from us. The key is to change our mindset. A new vision of health and well-being is emerging. Along with sustainability, resilience, deep ecology, and Gaia, we must embrace an inclusive and holistic concept of well-being.

The idea of 'well-being' has often been narrowly interpreted and poorly understood. It has been linked to personal growth and development; seeking job satisfaction, work/life balance, more time for yoga, walking, gardening, and resting. But this view is changing.

So, let's make it a global slogan: "I have the right to keep myself fit."

Your brain, which is at least 75 percent water and is like a soft-boiled egg, contains about 100 billion nerve cells, called neurons, seamlessly arranged and suspended in this aqueous environment. Each neuron resembles a leafless but elastic oak tree, with wiggly branches and root systems that connect and disconnect to other neurons. The number of connections a particular neuron makes ranges from 1,000 to more than 100,000, depending on its location in the brain. For example, your neocortex—your thinking brain—has about 10,000 to 40,000 connections per neuron.

We used to think of the brain as a computer, and while there are similarities, we now know there's much more to the story. Each neuron is a unique biocomputer, with more than 60 megabytes of RAM, capable of processing enormous amounts of data—up to hundreds of thousands of functions per second. As we learn new things and have new experiences, our neurons make new connections, exchanging electrochemical information with each other.

These connections are called synaptic connections because the place where the cells exchange information—the gap between the branch of one neuron and the root of another — is called the synapse.

As the brain makes these changes, our thoughts produce various chemicals called neurotransmitters (serotonin, dopamine, and acetylcholine are a few examples). When we think, neurotransmitters at one branch of one neuron cross the synaptic gap to reach the root of another neuron. Once they cross that gap, the neuron fires with an electrical bolt of information. When we continue thinking the same thoughts, the neuron keeps firing in the same ways, strengthening the relationship between the two cells so they can more readily convey a signal the next time those neurons fire.

As a result, the brain shows physical evidence that something was not only learned but also remembered. This process of selective strengthening is called synaptic potentiation. When clusters of neurons fire together to support a new thought, an additional chemical (a protein) is created within the nerve cell and makes its way to the cell's center, or nucleus, where it lands in the DNA. The protein then switches on several genes. Since the job of genes is to make proteins that maintain both the structure and function of the body, the nerve cell quickly makes a new protein to create new branches between nerve cells.

So when we repeat a thought or an experience enough times, our brain cells make not only stronger connections between each other (affecting our physiological functions) but also a greater number of total connections, which affects the physical structure of the body.

The brain becomes more enriched microscopically. As soon as you think a new thought, you change — neurologically, chemically, and genetically. In fact, you can gain thousands of new connections in seconds from novel learning, new ways of thinking, and fresh experiences.

This means that by thought alone, you can activate new genes right away.

So, after understanding these fascinating facts about how the brain works — which affects both mind and body — we can start thinking in new ways.

That is, "I am rising as the healthiest person in the world!"

Over time, mystical things will start happening with your body to make you healthy and fit.

As being healthy is our birthright, why not change the mindset to feel and think healthy?

Over time, your brain will do the work for you!

Chapter 3.3   How placebo can make you feel disease free as everything is in our mind

Suggestibility is a very loose term. You may not be the sort of person who responds well to a hypnotist on stage, but you might find, for example, that a doctor administering a placebo to you is something you respond well to.

<u>Derren Brown</u>

Most of us have heard about the "placebo." A placebo is anything that seems like a "real" medical treatment but isn't. It could be a pill, a shot, or some other type of "fake" treatment. What all placebos have in common is that they do not contain an active substance meant to affect health.

Have you ever tried a placebo in a real sense? Let's experience it. Would you like to taste an amazing energy drink?

In an empty Coca-Cola bottle, pour fresh drinking water and paste a label on the bottle side as "energy drink." Just look at the label for some time and then drink the water. If you do it convincingly, you will feel like you're having a real energy drink. That's the placebo effect.

Historically, it was standard practice for doctors to treat patients with a placebo to console them rather than to treat their symptoms. It wasn't until 1799 that the English physician John Haygarth pinpointed what was going on. Haygarth published his findings in a book called "On the Imagination as a Cause or as a Cure of Disorders of the Body," in which he wrote, "What a powerful influence upon diseases is produced by mere imagination."

The placebo effect gained further attention during World War II. When a badly injured American soldier was brought to the medical tent, Henry K. Beecher, an American anaesthesiologist, declared that he had to operate immediately. But in the war zone, there was a medical crisis, and there was no morphine available. If operated on without morphine, the pain alone could kill the soldier. One of Dr. Beecher's nurses had a bizarre idea. She filled a hypodermic needle with saline solution and told the soldier it was morphine. As soon as she injected the soldier, he began to relax. His pain subsided, and Dr. Beecher was able to operate successfully. That's the placebo effect!

Do you know the scientific basis of the placebo effect? No one exactly knows how it works, though a lot of research is ongoing. Research shows that the placebo effect creates a physical change in brain activity. A study conducted by the University of California, Los Angeles, Neuropsychiatric Institute in 2002 compared three groups of patients. Two groups were given experimental antidepressants, and the third group was given a placebo. Each group's brain activity was measured after a few weeks with an EEG machine. Out of all patients who reported a positive effect, those given the placebo showed a greater increase in brain activity. The study showed that this increased brain activity was in a different part of the brain that had received the placebo. This led researchers to conclude that the brain was not being tricked by the placebo but responded to it uniquely.

While we know the placebo effect works, no one is sure how or why. But study after study provides evidence that the placebo effect is real. What makes it work? One's belief system. Placebos have been shown to produce measurable physiological changes, such as an increase in heart rate or blood pressure. However, illnesses that rely on the self-reporting of symptoms for measurement are most strongly influenced by placebos, such as depression, anxiety, irritable bowel syndrome (IBS), and chronic pain.

I think, unconsciously or unknowingly, we use placebos most of the time. My daughter was suffering from fever and body aches, and I told her to take this parasafe 500 and she would feel better immediately. After consuming the tablet, she felt better after some time. What worked? Only the tablet? No, in my opinion, the placebo effect was there if you pay attention to it.

There are some conditions in which a placebo can produce results even when people know they are taking a placebo. Studies show that placebos can affect conditions such as:

- Depression
- Pain
- Sleep disorders
- Irritable bowel syndrome
- Menopause

Research on the placebo effect has focused on the relationship between mind and body. One common theory is that the placebo effect is due to a person's expectations. If a person expects a pill to do something, it's possible that the body's own chemistry can cause effects similar to what a medication might have caused. Experts also say that there is a relationship between how strongly a person expects to have results and whether or not results occur. The stronger the feeling, the more likely it is that a person will experience positive effects.

So, why not use it in real situations? At least, we can use it during the consumption of medicine, thinking that the medicine is affecting our body, and watch the magical things that start happening.

How does it work? The placebo effect changes from individual to individual, and its strength varies from one disease to the next. The reasons for the influence of a placebo are not fully understood. Given the variation in response, it is likely that more than one mechanism is at work.

Below are four factors said to be involved in the placebo effect:

1. **Expectation and conditioning:** Part of the power of the placebo lies in the expectations of the individual taking them. These

expectations can relate to the treatment, the substance, or the prescribing doctor. This expectation may cause a drop in stress hormones or cause them to recategorize their symptoms. For instance, a "sharp pain" might instead be perceived as an "uncomfortable tingling." On the other hand, if the individual does not expect the drug to work or expects side effects, the placebo can generate negative outcomes. In these cases, the placebo is referred to as a nocebo. In fact, the nocebo is more powerful than the placebo. One day, I was describing this to my wife. She laughed and didn't believe it. I did a demonstration. I asked her to focus her mind, concentrate on me, and listen to and feel my words very attentively. She laughed, but I told her that within a few minutes, she would feel nauseous. I told her to listen to my voice attentively, that within a few minutes, she would feel some indigestion in her stomach and she would vomit. She laughed it off. We both got busy with our daily routine. But after two hours, she told me that she was not feeling well, her stomach started behaving strangely, and she started vomiting. This is the nocebo effect.

2. **The placebo effect and the brain:** Brain imaging studies have found measurable changes in the neural activity of people experiencing placebo analgesia. Areas implicated include parts of the brain stem, spinal cord, nucleus accumbens, and amygdala. Strong placebo responses have also been linked to increases in dopamine and opioid receptor activity. Both chemicals are involved in reward and motivation pathways in the brain. Conversely, nocebos have been found to reduce dopamine and opioid receptor activity.

3. **Psychoneuroimmunology:** This is a relatively new area of scientific study that looks at the direct effect of brain activity on the immune system. Just as a dog can be conditioned to salivate at the sound of a bell, so can mice be conditioned to restrain their immune system when presented with a specific stimulus. It has long been known that a positive outlook can help stave off illness. In recent years, this pseudo-science has become scientific fact. Expecting

improvements in health can impact the efficacy of an individual's immune system. So, we must keep saying, "My immune system is becoming stronger and stronger."

4. **Evolved health regulation:** One explanation for the placebo effect is the evolution of the human brain's ability to moderate healing. The body of a mammal has developed helpful physiological responses to pathogens. For instance, fever helps remove bacteria and viruses by raising the internal temperature. However, as these responses come at a cost, the brain decides when to carry out a certain response. For example, in late pregnancy or during states of malnutrition, the body does not carry out the fever response to infection because a raised temperature could harm a baby or use up more energy than a starving individual can spare.

So, be the placebo! Next time you are not feeling well, just say and feel that every neuron, every cell in your body is getting strengthened and rejuvenated. This is what I do every time I feel unwell. After a certain period, I start to feel better!

Chapter3.4   How learning the basics of panic attacks can avert an impending cardiac problem

If we can soften our hearts, and if we can access the pure and simple aspect of our nature, then we can regain the realization that everything we need is already inside us and anything is attainable.

Yehuda Berg

When our son was enrolled in a residential school hostel in Guwahati, Assam, for Class XI, the hostel's stringent rules meant he had no contact with us for an entire month. The only exception was a brief, supervised phone call allowed every Sunday. After that month, we visited him and found that although he was physically fine, he felt trapped and likened the hostel to a jail due to the confined space and limited freedom.

Two months into his stay, we received an urgent call from the warden late at night, informing us that our son needed to be hospitalized. We rushed to the hospital and found him in bed, connected to an oxygen mask and an IV drip. His pulse had dropped to 35. Fortunately, after two IV drips, his condition stabilized, and he was discharged the next day. The doctor attributed his symptoms to the hostel's restrictive environment. Despite counselling, we decided to re-enrol him, but within three days, the same issue recurred, and he was hospitalized again.

This time, extensive tests were conducted, revealing a heart condition that necessitated surgery. However, seeking a second opinion in Gurgaon's Vedanta Hospital, further tests showed no heart issues. The doctor suggested that these episodes might be sporadic and advised letting him live normally. The incidents seemed linked to his stay in the hostel, prompting us to keep him at home for two months.

During this period, we sought counselling and identified the problem as panic attacks triggered by the hostel environment. Understanding the role of the amygdala in anxiety, we learned about two neural pathways responsible for anxiety: the cortex and the amygdala pathways. The cortex pathway deals with thoughts and logic, while the amygdala pathway triggers physical responses to fear. The amygdala reacts faster than the cortex, often causing symptoms like rapid heart rate, muscle tension, and adrenaline surges without conscious awareness.

Our son's panic attacks were triggered by the amygdala's fight-or-flight response. Recognizing this, we explained the amygdala's functions to him, helping him understand his reactions. We taught him coping strategies like deep breathing, muscle relaxation, and exercise to manage his anxiety. These techniques helped him calm down and reduce the duration of panic attacks.

We emphasized the importance of facing anxiety-inducing situations rather than avoiding them. By staying in the situation and using these techniques, he could retrain his amygdala to perceive the hostel environment as safe. This approach proved effective. After implementing these strategies, our son returned to the hostel and completed the next year and a half without any further panic attacks. Remarkably, he not only adapted well but also lost weight, becoming healthier and more resilient.

In conclusion, our son's journey through managing panic attacks in a challenging environment taught us the importance of understanding the brain's role in anxiety. By facing his fears and using effective coping strategies, he emerged stronger, healthier, and ready to tackle future challenges.

Chapter 4.1   Breathing is birth right and how it can help us to regain health issues

Whenever I feel blue, I start breathing again.

L. Frank Baum

Over the last one and a half months, we Indians have noticed a sharp increase in Covid-19 cases. Tragically, many people are dying. However, the most pressing issue highlighted is the severe shortage of hospital beds and oxygen supplies.

Yes, an oxygen crisis!

The shortage of life-saving oxygen cylinders has become a critical situation in India. As you may know, oxygen deficiency in Covid-19 patients can lead to severe conditions, such as:

- Severe pneumonia,
- Acute respiratory distress syndrome,
- Sepsis.

According to clinical management protocols, when the body is deprived of adequate oxygen at the tissue level, oxygen therapy is the primary treatment. This therapy aims to achieve 92-96%

SpO2, or 88-92% in patients with chronic obstructive pulmonary disease. If respiratory distress and hypoxemia persist despite standard oxygen therapy, high-flow nasal cannula oxygen therapy or non-invasive ventilation is recommended.

The goal of these treatments is to maintain the minimum oxygen intake necessary for survival. Oxygen intake is essential for survival!

Most Covid-19 patients suffer from respiratory tract infections, and in the most severe cases, symptoms include shortness of breath, potentially progressing to Acute Respiratory Distress Syndrome (ARDS). Thus, oxygen intake becomes vital.

Examining the situation, it's clear how crucial oxygen is for Covid-19 patients. But is it only for severely affected patients? Not at all. Oxygen is vital for everyone's survival, inhaled with every breath we take. It's such a natural process that we often forget it.

How many of us consciously practice deep breathing? Very few, I suspect. In this critical Covid-19 pandemic, when people are desperately seeking oxygen cylinders to save their loved ones, we should consider how deep breathing can help us. Deep breathing can maintain our oxygen intake, a practice we should have been aware of before the pandemic struck. Why wait until conditions worsen?

Breathing is our constant survival mode. By practicing deep breathing consciously, we can oxygenate our bodies and maintain a healthy bloodstream, lymphatic, and immune system.

The lymphatic system is crucial for overall health and immunity, yet few people are knowledgeable about it, and even fewer healthcare practitioners discuss it. The lymphatic system includes the bone marrow, tonsils, adenoids, spleen, thymus, lymph nodes, and lymphatic vessels. It works in partnership with the blood circulatory and immune systems to ward off infections, viruses, injury, and even cancer.

The lymphatic system can be thought of as the body's sewage system. Every cell is surrounded by lymph, which removes toxins and excess fluid. This system should be fully functional to keep us healthy. Unlike the heart in the blood circulatory system, the lymphatic system doesn't have an active pump and relies on muscular movement through exercise and deep breathing.

Exercise requires motivation and effort, but breathing is constant. By converting shallow breathing into deep breathing, we can oxygenate our bodies and maintain effective lymph and immune systems.

If the lymphatic system shuts down for just 24 hours, our toxin levels will rise, preventing oxygenation and leading to death. This is what happens in the current Covid-19 crisis — shortness of breath and oxygen.

The solution? Practice deep breathing!

Many people breathe shallowly, a habit formed by suppressing strong emotions. This shallow breathing keeps the body in a state of stress and can lead to various problems. Proper breathing, or deep diaphragmatic breathing, involves filling the lungs deeply and using the diaphragm.

Observe a newborn's breathing: they naturally practice deep breathing. As we age, we forget this and revert to shallow breathing. German philosopher Friedrich Nietzsche said, "In every real man a child is hidden that wants to play." Let us awaken the child within and start deep breathing.

Deep breathing involves the diaphragm's contraction, which pulls air into the lungs. Dr. Jack W. Shields' study showed that deep diaphragmatic breathing significantly stimulates lymph flow, more so than walking or jogging.

Starting today, commit to making deep breathing a lifestyle. Fight Covid-19 and rise as healthy individuals! Practice deep breathing with a ratio of 1:4:2, like a doctor's prescription. This means inhaling through the nose for one count, holding for four counts to distribute oxygen, and exhaling slowly for two counts. For example, inhale for five seconds, hold for twenty seconds, and exhale for ten seconds.

If practiced ten times each in the morning, noon, and evening, you will see considerable health improvements over time. Like the movie ABCD - Any Body Can Dance, anybody can breathe consciously to become a healthier person!

Chapter 4.2   Walking is most powerful alternative to every day exercise

If you're walking down the right path and you're willing to keep walking, eventually you'll make progress.

Barack Obama

Maintaining one's health and fitness is actually quite simple. However, over time, we tend to complicate things and become so hard on ourselves that we forget to utilize the simple, free tool that's always available to us and essential for life: breathing. Often, we neglect to do it consciously and deliberately, merely passing through life without paying much attention to it in terms of health.

Do you remember the moment you, as a baby or toddler, took your first shaky step or sprinted across the living room? Probably not. Yet, many of us vividly recall the excitement of watching a toddler's first steps, despite their unsteady legs. Those first steps, though not picture-perfect, leave an indelible mark on our memories.

As time passes and with practice, children—including you—begin to walk with their toes and feet turned at an angle. This gradual evolution from crawling to confident walking is a fundamental milestone in a child's development. Yet, as we transition from babies to adults, we often take walking for granted and forget that it's one of the best free tools for maintaining overall health.

Walking for the first time is one of the most exciting and memorable milestones in a child's development. From rolling, sitting up, bottom shuffling, crawling, and cruising along furniture, these activities build the muscle strength and coordination needed for walking. Parents closely observe these milestones, though they become routine and unremarkable as we age.

Initially, a baby needs to develop skills such as balance, coordination, and the ability to support their body weight from one leg to the other. Each new skill builds on the previous ones, becoming more complex over time. While busy crawling and pulling up to stand, babies build valuable muscle strength and coordination needed for walking and, later, running.

Some parents experience anxiety if their baby isn't walking by 18 months. It's important to understand different walking styles, such as in-toeing (feet turning inward) and out-toeing (feet pointing outward). Unfortunately, as we grow older, we often forget the struggle and effort involved in learning to walk. We overlook walking as a free and effective form of exercise.

Walking, a simple yet powerful activity, is one of the best forms of regular exercise. Have you ever considered its significance seriously? If not, what are you waiting for? By the end of this chapter, I hope you'll join the billions worldwide who have made walking a part of their daily routine. Some call it "Walk for Life," while others aim for "10,000 steps a day."

The number of steps you take each day indicates whether you're getting enough physical activity to reduce health risks and improve fitness. You can monitor your step count using a pedometer, fitness band, or mobile app. Don't settle for average. Increase your steps to reduce inactivity and achieve 30 minutes of exercise each day.

Have you ever made a commitment to yourself? Knowing how many steps you take daily can motivate you to join the global movement of 10,000 steps per day. This goal, though not originally based on research, has become a benchmark for moderate activity, supported by research from Catrine Tudor-Locke.

Are you still waiting? Join the global club of 10,000 steps per day! To stay motivated, consider the significance of walking in human history. A fossil foot bone from an early human ancestor, discovered in Hadar, Ethiopia, suggests that Australopithecus afarensis, a species from 3.2 million years ago, may have been the first human ancestor to walk upright.

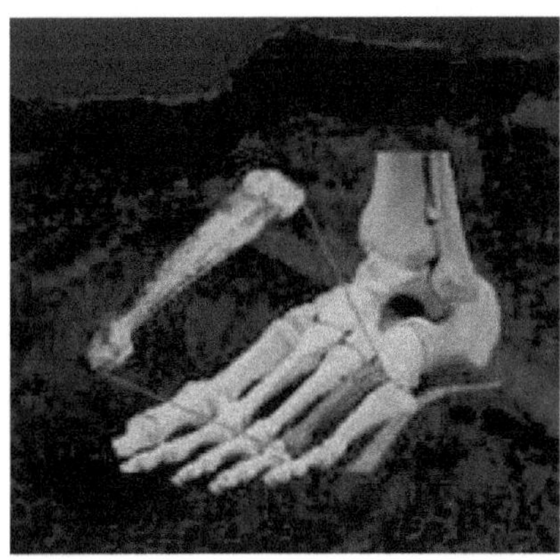

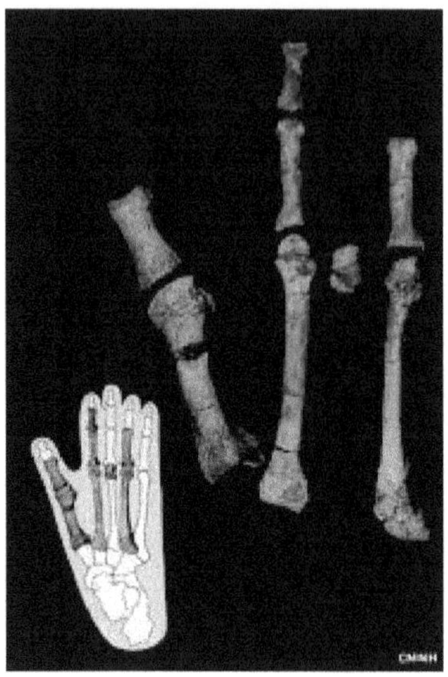

This discovery underscores the profound role of walking in human evolution.

So, let's walk together on this journey to better health and fitness!

In a recently published paper in *Science*, a team of anthropologists from the United States and Ethiopia described a newly discovered fossil as a fourth metatarsal, or mid-foot bone. This is the first such fossil ever found for *Australopithecus afarensis*, revealing that these ancient hominids had stiff, arched feet similar to humans, which enabled them to walk like us.

Australopithecus afarensis fossils were first discovered in Ethiopia in 1974. One of the best-known representatives of this species, also found in Hadar, was Lucy.

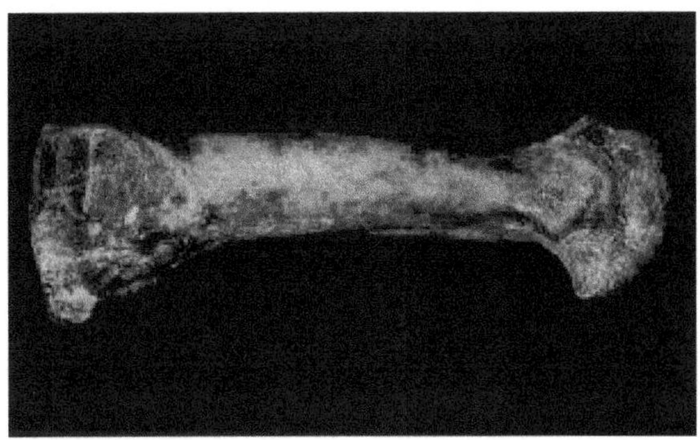

Of course, we're not talking about the character from the famous Hollywood movie *Lucy*. The name was given to several hundred bone pieces that made up about forty percent of one individual, believed to be female. There was significant controversy about whether Lucy and her relatives were strictly bipedal or if they also climbed trees. The discovery of this mid-foot bone has likely resolved those questions.

Knowing that Lucy and her relatives had arches in their feet impacts our understanding of many aspects of their lives, from their habitat to their diet and their strategies for avoiding predators. The development of arched feet was a crucial step toward the human condition, as it signified the abandonment of the ability to use the big toe for grasping branches, indicating that our ancestors had left the trees for life on the ground.

Arches in the feet are essential for human-like walking because they absorb shock and provide a stiff platform to push off from, facilitating forward movement. Today, people with flat feet, who lack arches, often suffer from various joint problems throughout their bodies. Understanding that the arch appeared early in our evolution underscores the importance of this unique structure for human locomotion.

Recognizing what our ancestors were designed to do and the natural selection that shaped the human skeleton offers insights into how our skeletons function today. The significance of arches in our feet was as vital for our ancestors as it is for us — for walking!

We can only imagine what life was like for Lucy and her kind. They were small-statured, possibly covered in fur, with males just under five feet tall and weighing under 100 pounds, while females were about three and a half feet tall and 60 pounds. Their brains were smaller than ours, and they had powerful jaws for eating leaves, seeds, roots, fruit, nuts, and insects. With the discovery of this fossil foot bone, we now know they had arched feet, much like ours. They were likely the first in the evolutionary path toward being human to walk upright through the ancient forests and open lands of Ethiopia, foraging for food.

Visualize this: our ancestors had arched feet similar to ours, which they used to walk and run for their very survival. How much do we know about our feet, which we now underutilize due to our sedentary lifestyles? The result? Look around—numerous health problems, including depression, anxiety, and a tendency toward suicide.

The foot is the lowest point of the human leg, and its shape, along with the body's natural balance-keeping systems, enables humans to walk, run, climb, and perform countless other activities.

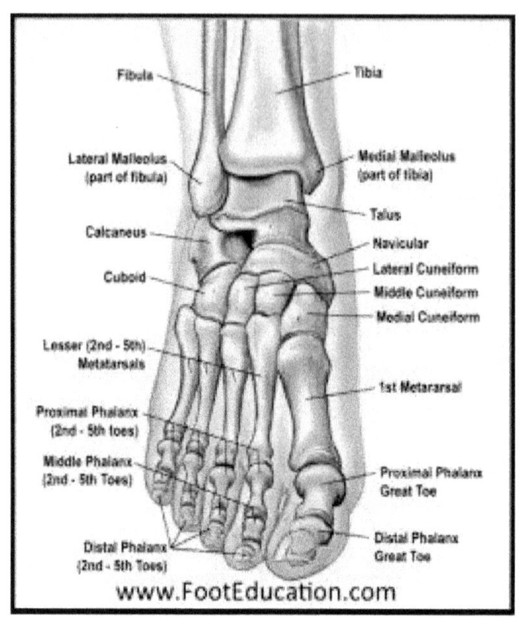

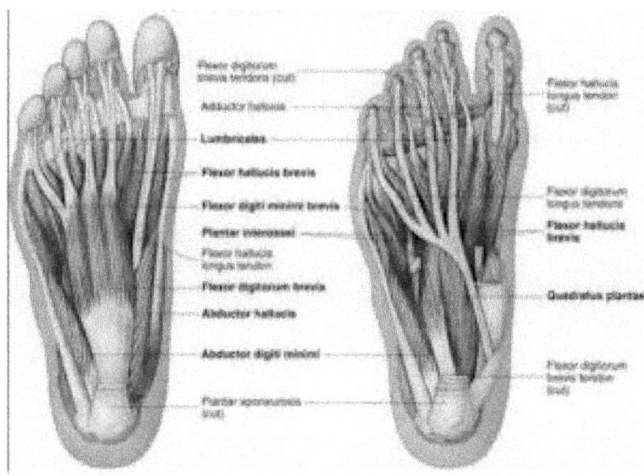

The foot's complex structure includes more than 100 tendons, ligaments, and muscles that move nearly three dozen joints, while bones provide structure. The foot is similar to the hand but is stronger and less mobile due to bearing more weight.

The largest bone in the foot, the calcaneus, forms the heel, which slopes upward to meet the tarsal bones that point downward with the remaining foot bones. Below these bones are the foot's arches — the medial arch, lateral arch, and fundamental longitudinal arch — which make walking easier and less taxing. These arches are created by the angles of the bones and strengthened by the tendons and ligaments connecting the bones.

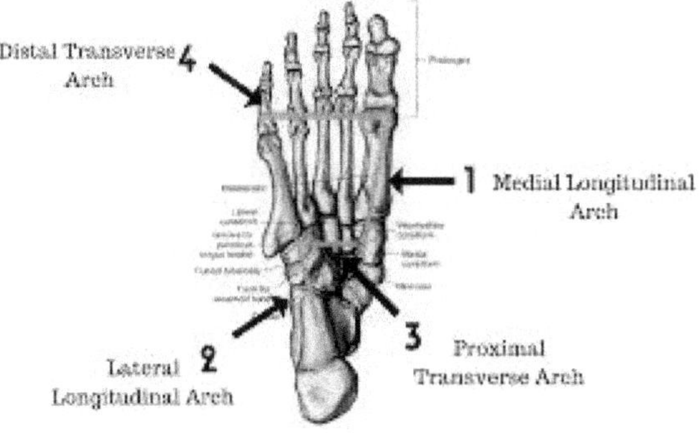

The bones of the foot are organized into rows named tarsal bones, metatarsal bones, and phalanges, making up the toes and the broad section of the feet. Walking can help lower your risk of heart disease, cancer, diabetes, and blood pressure, and cholesterol levels, and even keep your memory sharp.

You've probably heard the phrase, "To walk is to be human." We're the only species that moves by standing up and putting one foot in front of the other. In the six million years humans have been bipedal, our ability to walk upright has allowed us to travel great distances and survive changing climates, environments, and landscapes. Yet, many of us ignore walking as a beneficial exercise.

Countless scientific studies have shown that walking can provide numerous health benefits, helping us stay healthy. The beauty of walking is that it's free, doesn't require special equipment, and can be done almost anywhere, making it an excellent form of regular exercise. Most people can maintain a walking practice throughout their lives.

Now, let's return to the global club of "Walk 10,000 Steps a Day." Do you really need it? Interestingly, this recommendation didn't originate from science but from a 1960s advertising campaign to promote a pedometer in Japan. Despite its origins, the campaign gained popularity, and countries like the U.S. have included it in broader public health recommendations. Today, it's a default step count goal on many walking apps and fitness trackers.

Since the 1960s, researchers have studied the 10,000-step-a-day standard with mixed results. Do you know the average steps an Indian takes per day? It's only 4,297 steps—much less than the 10,000-step goal. This equates to 2.15 miles or 3.44 kilometers per day. The result? Numerous health issues in our country, exacerbated by the COVID-19 pandemic.

The average number of steps per day varies by country due to factors such as obesity rates, climate, walkability of roads and sidewalks, and income. To put yourself on track with walking, remember why it's so important. For instance, a recent Harvard study involving more than 16,000 older women found that those who took at least 4,400 steps a day greatly reduced their risk of dying prematurely compared to less active women. The longevity benefits continued up to 7,500 steps but leveled off after that number. Therefore, 7,500 steps a day is also an ideal goal with comparable benefits to 10,000 steps.

The rule of thumb is to get at least 150 minutes of moderate-intensity aerobic exercise a week, according to the 2018 Physical Activity Guidelines for Americans. Fascinatingly, a study from the University of Utah showed that the body may actually be made to walk. Walking is physically easier on the body but still requires taking in more oxygen than in a sedentary mode, providing the same benefits as running. It's easy to forget that walking is an aerobic activity.

That's why about 7 billion people do it every day — because walking is the best form of regular exercise. The amount you walk, rather than how fast you walk, might be more important for reducing cancer mortality, as studies have noted.

So, from today onwards, commit to walking. Taking more steps each day will make a significant difference in the coming days. Remember, our goal is to rise as healthy individuals!

Chapter 4.3   Fasting is good for overall health

Fasting is, first and foremost, an exercise for identifying and managing adversity in all its forms. With faith, in full conscience, fasting calls women and men to an extra degree of self-awareness.

Tariq Ramadan

As Muslims, we are called to practice deliberate fasting. Initially, we engage in this practice from a religious perspective, fulfilling a spiritual duty. However, my understanding of fasting deepened when I encountered the groundbreaking work of Japanese cell biologist Yoshinori Ohsumi. In 2016, Ohsumi won the Nobel Prize in Medicine for his research on autophagy, the process by which cells recycle and renew their content.

Ohsumi's research revealed that fasting activates autophagy, a critical process for cell health, renewal, and survival. During periods of starvation, cells break down proteins and other components for energy. This process allows cells to destroy viruses and bacteria and eliminate damaged structures. Ohsumi's work, primarily conducted in yeast, showed that autophagy genes are also present in higher organisms, including humans, and that mutations in these genes can lead to disease. Autophagy is essential for animals, plants, and single-cell organisms to survive famines.

Although the concept of autophagy was discovered in the 1960s, Ohsumi's research from the late 1980s onwards demonstrated its role in protecting against inflammation and diseases like dementia and Parkinson's. His pioneering efforts created a new field of science, transforming the understanding of cellular processes. When Ohsumi began his research, fewer than 20 papers on autophagy were published annually; today, more than 5,000 papers are published each year, spanning diverse fields including cancer and longevity studies.

Fasting has been a part of religious, spiritual, and health practices throughout human history. In the blue zones region of Ikaria, known for its long-living inhabitants, people observe about 150 days of religious fasting each year. Scientists have found that fasting for 12 to 24 hours triggers autophagy, which is believed to be one reason fasting is associated with longevity.

The health benefits of intermittent fasting are well-documented. Here are ten evidence-based benefits:

1. **Changes the Function of Hormones, Cells, and Genes**: During fasting, hormone levels shift to make stored body fat more accessible, and essential cellular repair processes are initiated. Insulin levels drop significantly, facilitating fat burning. Human growth hormone (HGH) levels increase, promoting fat burning and muscle gain. Cellular repair processes remove waste material from cells, and beneficial changes occur in genes related to longevity and disease protection.

2. **Weight Loss and Reduction of Visceral Fat**: Intermittent fasting typically leads to fewer meals consumed, resulting in a lower caloric intake. Enhanced hormone function further supports weight loss.

3. **Reduced Insulin Resistance and Lower Risk of Type 2 Diabetes**: Intermittent fasting can decrease insulin resistance, helping to lower blood sugar levels and protect against type 2 diabetes.

4. **Reduced Oxidative Stress and Inflammation**: Fasting reduces oxidative stress, a factor in aging and chronic diseases.

This involves the reduction of free radicals, which can damage proteins and DNA.

One particularly inspiring example is our colleague, Barman, who started fasting every Thursday after learning about these tremendous health benefits. He has maintained this practice for the past year and is committed to continuing it for the rest of his life.

Fasting, therefore, is not just a religious obligation but also a scientifically validated practice that promotes health and longevity. By understanding and embracing the benefits of fasting, we can enhance our spiritual well-being and our physical health.

Chapter 4.4   Know your telomere to regain health issues

The journey is never-ending. There's always gonna be growth, improvement, adversity; you just gotta take it all in and do what's right, continue to grow, continue to live in the moment.

Anonymous

How many of us truly believe that we can reverse aging? Imagine living longer than we ever thought possible. Sounds cool, right? Yes, it is! While we all have to face mortality someday, why not embrace the latest breakthroughs in medical science to help us combat aging? For the time we have, why not live younger, more agile, and full of vitality — without noticeable disease?

I bet everyone reading this is nodding in agreement. Imagine a life with a longer health span and a shorter disease span. Our goal should be to extend our health span, living a long, healthy life until the very end. To achieve this, we must understand our biology at the cellular level. Did you know that cellular aging begins in the womb? Yes, aging starts in utero!

Enter the telomere effect. Telomeres are the ends of chromosomes, made of repetitive DNA sequences that protect chromosomes from damage. Each time a cell divides, telomeres shorten, eventually becoming too short for the cell to divide further. This leads to aging and cellular degradation. Understanding telomeres is crucial for anti-aging.

Telomeres act like caps on the ends of chromosomes, preventing them from fraying or tangling during replication. Hermann Muller first identified these unique chromosome ends in the 1930s, coining the term "telomeres" from Greek words meaning "end" and "part." Shortened telomeres are linked to aging diseases like heart disease, cancer, and osteoporosis. The longer the telomeres, the longer the lifespan and the healthier the cells.

In India, you can get your telomere length tested at DNA labs, which offer a Telomere Age Test across 3,000 sample collection centers. This test helps you understand your biological aging and take steps to improve your telomere length.

Telomerase is an enzyme that repairs telomeres. Without enough telomerase, our bodies struggle to maintain telomere length. Remember the movie "Pa," where Amitabh Bachchan plays a child with progeria, a genetic disorder that accelerates aging? While we don't face such extreme aging, factors like chronic stress, chemical exposure, and poor living conditions can shorten our telomeres.

Research published in *Nature* showed that mice without telomerase aged prematurely but became younger when telomerase was reintroduced. This demonstrates that we have more control over our telomeres than previously thought. While we can't change the telomeres inherited from our parents, we can lengthen them with lifestyle changes.

To slow down aging and live healthier, start by managing stress. Stress is unavoidable, but chronic stress shortens telomeres. Approach stress with resilience to protect your telomeres. Make exercise a daily habit. Moderate cardiovascular exercise and high-intensity interval training reduce oxidative stress and inflammation, benefiting telomeres. Maintain a healthy weight; excess body fat accelerates telomere shortening.

Your diet plays a crucial role. Avoid high-sugar diets and focus on whole foods like vegetables, fruits, whole grains, nuts, legumes, and omega-3 fatty acids. These foods reduce oxidative stress, inflammation, and insulin resistance, benefiting telomeres. Finally, consider supplements like vitamin D, which is linked to longer telomere length. Consult your doctor before starting any supplements.

The groundbreaking research by Dr. Elizabeth Blackburn and Dr. Elissa Epel on telomeres offers a new understanding of health and longevity. By understanding and taking action on our telomere health, we can slow down aging and live longer, healthier lives

Chapter 5.1   Acknowledging and accepting how your present biological age is the key to go to the next level.

Every child should have a caring adult in their lives. And that's not always a biological parent or family member. It may be a friend or neighbour. Often it is a teacher.

Joe Manchin

How many of us truly believe that we can reverse aging? Imagine living longer than we ever thought possible. Sounds cool, right? Yes, it is! While we all have to face mortality someday, why not embrace the latest breakthroughs in medical science to help us combat aging? For the time we have, why not live younger, more agile, and full of vitality — without noticeable disease?

I bet everyone reading this is nodding in agreement. Imagine a life with a longer health span and a shorter disease span. Our goal should be to extend our health span, living a long, healthy life until the very end. To achieve this, we must understand our biology at the cellular level. Did you know that cellular aging begins in the womb? Yes, aging starts in utero!

Enter the telomere effect. Telomeres are the ends of chromosomes, made of repetitive DNA sequences that protect chromosomes from damage. Each time a cell divides, telomeres shorten, eventually becoming too short for the cell to divide further. This leads to aging and cellular degradation. Understanding telomeres is crucial for anti-aging.

Telomeres act like caps on the ends of chromosomes, preventing them from fraying or tangling during replication. Hermann Muller first identified these unique chromosome ends in the 1930s, coining the term "telomeres" from Greek words meaning "end" and "part." Shortened telomeres are linked to aging diseases like heart disease, cancer, and osteoporosis. The longer the telomeres, the longer the lifespan and the healthier the cells.

In India, you can get your telomere length tested at DNA labs, which offer a Telomere Age Test across 3,000 sample collection centers. This test helps you understand your biological aging and take steps to improve your telomere length.

Telomerase is an enzyme that repairs telomeres. Without enough telomerase, our bodies struggle to maintain telomere length. Remember the movie "Pa," where Amitabh Bachchan plays a child with progeria, a genetic disorder that accelerates aging? While we don't face such extreme aging, factors like chronic stress, chemical exposure, and poor living conditions can shorten our telomeres.

Research published in *Nature* showed that mice without telomerase aged prematurely but became younger when telomerase was reintroduced. This demonstrates that we have more control over our telomeres than previously thought. While we can't change the telomeres inherited from our parents, we can lengthen them with lifestyle changes.

To slow down aging and live healthier, start by managing stress. Stress is unavoidable, but chronic stress shortens telomeres. Approach stress with resilience to protect your telomeres. Make exercise a daily habit. Moderate cardiovascular exercise and high-intensity interval training reduce oxidative stress and inflammation, benefiting telomeres. Maintain a healthy weight; excess body fat accelerates telomere shortening.

Your diet plays a crucial role. Avoid high-sugar diets and focus on whole foods like vegetables, fruits, whole grains, nuts, legumes, and omega-3 fatty acids. These foods reduce oxidative stress, inflammation, and insulin resistance, benefiting telomeres. Finally, consider supplements like vitamin D, which is linked to longer telomere length. Consult your doctor before starting any supplements.

The groundbreaking research by Dr. Elizabeth Blackburn and Dr. Elissa Epel on telomeres offers a new understanding of health and longevity. By understanding and taking action on our telomere health, we can slow down aging and live longer, healthier lives

Chapter 5.2   More effective than physical activity is feeling well through visualization and affirmation.

Life is an affirmation, not defamation. Life means living. Life means taking that one tiny or giant leap beyond what you know you can do, or simply beyond what you know. It is in these moments that we live.

RickTumlinson

Forget "No pain, no gain." Scientists are proving that simply visualizing what you want can help make it a reality. Let's get one thing out of the way: No, fantasizing about Arnold Schwarzenegger isn't going to make him appear at your door. But imagining yourself sculpting sexy arms might just lead to definitive results. "Psychologists have known for decades that the images you create in your mind can have a potent effect on your body; now researchers are proving it," says Traci Stein, PhD, a clinical psychologist and adjunct professor at Columbia University's Teachers College in New York City.

It sounds woo-woo, yet mounting evidence shows that visualization works. For example, Cleveland Clinic scientists discovered that people who performed "mental contractions" of the abductor muscle in their little finger over 12 weeks increased its strength by 35 percent—not far from the boost in strength experienced by people who did actual little-finger exercises (53 percent). "Visualization activates the same neural networks that actual task performance does, which can strengthen the connection between brain and body," explains neuroscientist Stephen Kosslyn, PhD, author of *Top Brain, Bottom Brain*. Indeed, an MRI study in *The Journal of Neuroscience* found that whether people performed physical finger exercises or just imagined doing them, activity shot up in the part of their brain where nerve pulses initiate muscle movement.

"There's no question that this mental processing results in real-life improvement," adds Kosslyn. In the 2015 FIFA Women's World Cup Final, USA Soccer star Carli Lloyd credited visualization for her hat trick against Japan—that's three goals in a row! Besides helping you hit your targets, visualization has been linked to better sleep, less inflammation, and lower blood pressure and stress levels.

Here are a few easy ways you can use this Jedi mind trick to achieve almost anything you want:

See yourself getting in awesome shape: Research shows that "motivational general-mastery imagery"—in which you imagine yourself conquering that huge hill or kicking ass during the bike portion of your upcoming triathlon—may help you push your limits and thus get fitter. "This kind of positive visualization lets you eliminate nerves and self-doubt," explains Margaret Ottley, PhD, professor of sport and exercise psychology at West Chester University of Pennsylvania. Use it to tack an extra mile onto your run by picturing yourself sailing past your usual turnoff point.

Picture yourself stronger: "Building physical strength is more than just accumulating muscle mass," says Brian Clark, PhD, professor of physiology and neuroscience at Ohio University. "Visualization enhances neural pathways in your brain so it's easier for your nervous system to activate those muscles in real life." Clark studied volunteers who wore an elbow-to-finger cast for four weeks. Half of those people did a mental wrist workout (they visualized themselves flexing their wrist muscles) five days a week. The other half did nothing. At the end of the study, the folks in the first group had lost 50 percent less strength. Next time you're at the gym, try using your breaks between sets to imagine yourself clenching your butt in a glute bridge or tightening your abs in a plank twist.

At the same time, positive affirmation can create a miraculous shift in our lives. Affirmations are positive reminders or statements that can be used to encourage and motivate yourself or others. Often it's easier to affirm others than it is ourselves, but we need to remember to encourage ourselves as well. Some people say affirmations out loud in front of a mirror. Others simply write them down in a journal. You can also repeat them in your head like a mantra during meditation. The important thing is to find affirmations that resonate with you. I'll admit that there are plenty of affirmations out there that are just too woo-woo for me and do not resonate with me. Sometimes people throw in words like "manifest" and "abundance," but these words simply don't resonate with me (but maybe they do for you!). The important thing is to find affirmations that resonate with you.

Start by choosing two to three affirmations from the list below that resonate with you. From there, decide if you will say them aloud, write them down, or recite them in your head. Try to do this in the morning or before you go to bed as part of your daily routine. The key here is that you don't have to go through a running list of affirmations every day. Just choose a few that speak to you and encourage you to keep moving forward. Self-affirmation encourages you to think positively about the important things in your life. Rather than trying to convince yourself that you're beautiful when you don't feel that way, self-affirmation encourages you to think positively about the important things in your life, like your health, family, career, or hobbies. This means reflecting on things that you know and believe are good about yourself and your life.

Daily Affirmations List to Improve Your Mindset: Here are some examples of affirmations that you can use daily. Pick a few that resonate with you or simply write your own!

1. I create a safe and secure space for myself wherever I am.
2. I permit myself to do what is right for me.
3. I am confident in my ability to make myself healthy and fit.
4. I feel proud of myself when I [fill in the blank].
5. I give myself space to grow and learn.

6. I allow myself to be who I am without judgment.

7. I give myself the care and attention that I deserve.

8. My drive and ambition allow me to achieve my goals.

9. I am creatively inspired by the world around me.

10. I am becoming closer to my true self every day.

11. I am grateful to have people in my life who inspire me to be healthy.

12. I am learning valuable lessons from myself every day.

13. I am at peace with who I am as a person.

14. I make a difference in the world by simply existing in it.

It might sound counterintuitive to combine visualization and meditation. After all, meditation is all about letting thoughts come and go rather than consciously directing them toward a particular result, right? When you visualize, you focus on something specific — an event, person, or goal you want to achieve — and hold it in your mind, imagining your outcome becoming reality. Visualization is a mindfulness technique on its own, but you can also use it to enhance regular meditation. Adding visualization into your meditation mix allows you to better direct your relaxed mind toward specific outcomes you'd like to see.

Plus, visualization is linked to many potential health benefits, including increased athletic performance, relief of anxiety and depression symptoms, improved relaxation, greater compassion for yourself and others, pain relief, improved ability to cope with stress, improved sleep, greater emotional and physical wellness, and increased self-confidence.

The consistent affirmation that the rise of a healthy person is in abundance will make the world a better place to live in.

Chapter 5.3   Quick fix to overcome stress and anxiety within seconds

Your body hears everything your mind says.

Naomi Judd

Fear can create strong signals of response when we're in emergencies – for instance, if we are caught in a fire or are being attacked. It can also take effect when you're faced with non-dangerous events, like exams, public speaking, a new job, a date, or even a party, or thinking that you may have some life-threatening disease. It's a natural response to a threat that can be either perceived or real. Stress and anxiety is a word we use for some types of fear that are usually to do with the thought of a threat or something going wrong in the future, rather than right now.

Fear and anxiety can last for a short time and then pass, but they can also last much longer and you can get stuck with them. In some cases, they can take over your life, affecting your ability to eat, sleep, concentrate, travel, enjoy life, or even leave the house or go to work or school. This can hold you back from doing things you want or need to do, and most importantly, it also affects your health. Some people become overwhelmed by fear and want to avoid situations that might make them frightened or anxious. It can be hard to break this cycle, but there are lots of ways to do it.

Once we know how our mind works, we can easily fix stress and anxiety more productively. As my wife suffers from common diseases like diabetes and high blood pressure which result from stress and anxiety, our main emphasis is how to deal with these stress and anxiety. As you may know, we perceive information through five senses- Visual (what we see), auditory (what we hear), kinaesthetic (what we feel), olfactory (what we smell), and gustatory (what we taste). Events or incidents we experience in our life go through three different phases that are Deletion, distortion, and generalisation and then it goes to our subconscious mind where it gets stored.

Specifically, stress or anxiety-generating events or incidents go to our permanent memory which we hardly forget and because of this, as we go into fight or flight or freeze mode, two hormones secrete from our brain: Cortisol and Adrenaline. Over time, as we use to remember those stressful or anxiety-producing events, these hormones secrete. Even though these two hormones are good for us, when we are in slow but consistent stress or anxiety because of our present lifestyle, these hormones are produced more and more.

Because of cortisol, sugar in the blood increases and over time we may become victims of diabetes. And, because of adrenaline, the heart needs to pump more blood which eventually makes our heart beat faster and when it happens again and again, we may become victims of high blood pressure. Now, coming back to my wife's suffering from diabetes and high blood pressure, it can easily be understood that because of constant stress and anxiety situations which we can't avoid most of the time and sometimes we have those unconsciously, we are at risk to develop diabetes and high blood pressure.

Each of the anxiety disorders above has its range of therapies and coping strategies. Many forms of anxiety can be successfully treated with psychological therapies such as Cognitive Behavioural Therapy (CBT), cognitive restructuring, or medication. There are also various techniques for managing some of the common symptoms of anxiety. These can be helpful when you're going through worrying times, at home or work, or facing particular challenges that make you anxious. Though you may be familiar with different strategies, sometimes refreshing your knowledge to cope with these six strategies can make a significant difference.

1. Identify Sources of Stress: Stress, particularly long-term stress, is strongly linked to anxiety. Another approach is to start keeping a stress diary. Every day, write down the stresses that you experience and record any anxious thoughts that you have. After a few days, read your diary and explore possible causes and triggers. Once you've identified specific sources of stress and anxiety, you can take steps to avoid them – or at least to manage your feelings toward them.

2. Exercise More: Studies show that regular exercise can help to reduce anxiety and build your stress tolerance. Yoga can be especially useful for managing anxiety since it helps to slow and focus your breathing, and can give you more control over your body and mind.

3. Watch What You Eat: You can often lessen your anxiety by reducing or avoiding certain foods and drinks. For example, consider limiting your intake of caffeine, alcohol, soda, energy drinks, and chocolate.

4. Use Relaxation Techniques: You can use deep breathing exercises to control your stress and anxiety. Deep breathing is especially effective for managing short-term anxiety.

5. Think Positively: Often, anxious episodes are preceded by self-sabotaging thoughts or behaviours. To help with this, write down any negative thoughts as soon as they arise. Then, note down the exact opposites of those thoughts. As you write out these positive affirmations, start to visualize successful outcomes – both what you hope to happen, and how you want to feel. Mentally rehearsing your meeting like this should relax your mind and body and help to keep your anxiety under control.

6. Get More Organized: Poor organization can be a serious source of stress and anxiety. If this is the case with you, you'll likely benefit from learning good time-management skills. Make sure that you manage your daily tasks and responsibilities effectively.

Do you want to apply a quick fix to vanish your stress and anxiety instantly? Then, do this:

This visualization technique can help with stress relief and general mood improvement. To start, think of something you want to bring into yourself. This could be a specific emotion or just positive vibes. Now, assign this feeling a colour. There's no right or wrong answer here, but consider choosing a colour you like or find soothing. Once you have your desired emotion and corresponding colour in mind, follow these steps:

1. Get comfortable, just as you would for ordinary meditation.
2. Close your eyes and relax by breathing slowly and deeply.
3. Visualize the colour you've chosen.
4. Continue breathing while holding that colour in your thoughts, thinking about what it represents for you.
5. With each inhale, imagine the desired colour slowly washing over your body from head to toe. Continue breathing as you visualize the colour filling your entire body, including your fingertips and toes.

6. Imagine any unwanted emotions draining out of your body with each exhale, and replace them with your chosen colour with each inhale.

7. Continue the visualization as long as you like. You might feel lightened and more peaceful after just a minute or two.

You can use colour breathing as part of any meditation, but you can also take a few moments for colour breathing even when you don't have time for a full meditation.

Chapter 5.4 Understanding heart intelligence and practicing heart coherence meditation makes the world a healthier place

Your time is limited, so don't waste it living someone else's life. Don't be trapped by dogma - which is living with the results of other people's thinking. Don't let the noise of others' opinions drown out your own inner voice. And most important, dare to follow your heart and intuition.

Steve Jobs

Have you ever heard the saying, "think with your heart, not your head"? This statement holds more meaning and scientific evidence now than ever before! The ability to study the heart has advanced tremendously in recent years, giving us a much better understanding of the greater role the heart plays, both within the operation of the body and our overall energetic well-being.

Traditionally, western science has described the brain as the epicenter, or sole location, where the body processes sensory input, comprehends the external world, and understands emotion. However, more and more research is showing us that the heart processes information through sensory neurons just like the brain does. The heart, like the brain, contains clusters of neurons that store short and long-term memory. These so-called "heart memories" are then sent to the brain to help manoeuvre our emotional experiences and guide our decision-making.

We once thought that the brain sent neural signals to inform the heart of its functions, but now we know… the heart sends more signals to the brain than it receives. The heart and brain are constantly having a two-way conversation. This knowledge provides a much more holistic model to help us understand and create clarity out of an ever-changing and overstimulating world. We also know that this is just the beginning of what modern science is revealing about matters of the heart.

Isn't it fascinating that quite often you can feel someone has entered the room before you see them? Or when you meet someone whom you feel wonderful around, and you just know their energy is good? The heart not only affects our internal functioning but also can influence the energy of those around us. How is this possible?

The heart has been measured to have an electromagnetic field that radiates up to 5-8 feet (2-

3 meters) around us in all directions. It is 100 times electrically stronger, and up to 5,000 times magnetically stronger, than the brain. This makes it the strongest electromagnetic force in the body.

The heart senses emotional information five to seven seconds before it happens, while the brain senses it three to five seconds beforehand. So not only are emotions important contributors to our output of thoughts, but they may be one of the best ways to influence and create a change in what and how we think.

In 1974, French researchers Gahery and Vigier stimulated the vagus nerve (which carries signals from the heart to the brain) in cats and found that the heart and nervous system were not simply following the brain's directions. In 1983, the heart was reclassified as an endocrine gland when a new hormone called atrial natriuretic factor (ANF), which affects blood vessels, kidneys, adrenal glands, and regulatory regions in the brain, was found to be produced by the heart.

Dr. J. Andrew Armour discovered the heart also contains a cell type known as intrinsic cardiac adrenergic (ICA), which synthesizes and releases neurotransmitters once thought to be produced only by neurons in the brain and nerve ganglia. The heart starts beating in an unborn fetus before the brain has been formed, a process scientists call "autorhythmic." Dr. Armour, a pioneer in this field, has undertaken extensive research and introduced the concept of the intrinsic cardiac network as a functional "heart brain." His work demonstrated a complex intrinsic nervous system in the heart, that is deemed sufficiently sophisticated to qualify as a "little brain" in its own right. With as many as 40,000 neurons, the heart is a nervous system that functions independently of the brain. The technical term coined for this system is the intrinsic cardiac system, more commonly known as the heart-brain.

These signals from the heart to the brain connect through the vagus nerve and continue straight to the thalamus, which synchronizes cortical activity such as thinking, perceiving, and understanding linguistics, then to the frontal lobes, which synchronize motor functions and problem-solving.

It is quite evident that when we become more heart-centered, we are least likely to react to stressors in our life. The reverse is also true. When we are not centered in our hearts, we are living in survival mode.

To enhance our heart-centeredness, we can practice heart coherence meditation developed by the USA's notable institute, HeartMath Institute. Here's how you can do it:

1. Close your eyes. Make yourself comfortable and relaxed.
2. Pay attention to the heart center. Start breathing in and out from the heart center, doing this more slowly and deeply.
3. When your mind wanders, keep returning your attention and awareness to your chest, to your heart, and your breath.
4. While you continuously put your attention to the heart, bring up some elevated emotions while continuing to breathe in and out of your heart center.
5. Once you feel these heartfelt emotions in your chest area, send the energy out beyond your body and marry it with your intention.
6. Continue to broadcast that energy and intention all around you. Start with 10 minutes and try to extend the time you practice every day. Eventually, you will

come to know what it feels like in your body to experience these elevated emotions. You can practice throughout your day with your eyes open. You might even set a reminder on your phone four times a day when it goes off, take a minute or two to feel those elevated emotions.

Not only because of the pandemic coronavirus, but overall, we are living in a time of extremes, and these extremes are the broader conception of old consciousness driven by survival emotions like hatred, violence, anger, fear, suffering, competition, and pain. We, as the human race, feel disconnected.

In this age of information, everything that is not in alignment with new consciousness is because we might not be paying attention to our own state of being and mankind's interconnectedness to this energy by focusing more on heart intelligence. As the heart is an independent intelligence radiating a strong electromagnetic field all around us, if we can meditate as described above with the clear intention of world peace and harmony, it affects the mass community at large, in addition to individual health.

The Global Coherence Initiative is a science-based, co-creative project to unite people in heart-focused love and intention, to facilitate the shift in global consciousness from instability and discord to compassionate care, cooperation, and increasing peace. Global coherence research encompasses a large variety of scientific data to gain new insights into the interconnectedness of human/animal health and behavior and the sun and earth's magnetic activity. The scientific community is just beginning to appreciate and understand the deeper level of how we are interconnected. We are getting closer to understanding why and how magnetic fields generated by the sun and earth affect human health and behavior – and why it is important to know this.

Let us make this world a better place by joining HeartMath Institute's Global Coherence Initiative. In a nutshell, when we do more and more heart-based meditation, we, as individuals, can not only rise as healthy persons but we can make the world community as a whole a better place to live in. This way, we can create a meaningful legacy for future generations, ensuring that the world we live in is not just the world we see today, but the best place on planet Earth to live in.

Chapter 5.5 How dance could be a major contributory factor for mental and physical health to rise as healthy person.

"I do not try to dance better than anyone else. I only try to dance better than myself."
Mikhail Baryshnikov

When I recently joined Tiru Sameer's online dance course, ACD, that is Anyone Can Dance ,my curiosity led me to a surprising revelation: dance offers incredible health benefits! In his introductory speech, Sameer enlightened us about DOSE— Dopamine, Oxytocin, Serotonin, and Endorphins, the four crucial hormones that dance helps release. That moment struck me like a lightbulb.

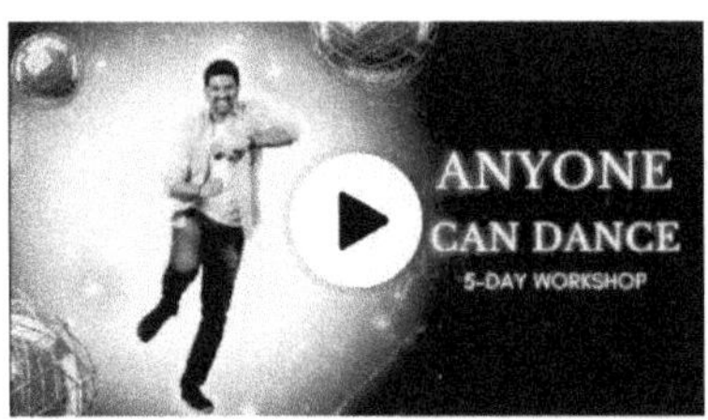

You've likely heard of these happy hormones: Serotonin, Dopamine, Endorphins, and Oxytocin. They are vital for promoting happiness and pleasure while reducing depression and anxiety. Engaging in simple activities can naturally boost these feel-good hormones, and dance is a major contributor.

People might laugh, thinking I'm too old to start dancing, but I say, "Yes, you should!" Dance helps release DOSE. Here's what each hormone does for us:

- **Dopamine**: Integral to the brain's reward system, it helps us feel pleasure and influences learning, attention, mood, movement, heart rate, kidney function, blood vessel function, sleep, pain processing, and lactation.

- **Oxytocin**: Produced in the hypothalamus and released by the pituitary gland, it's often called the "love hormone" because it facilitates childbirth. It decreases stress and anxiety, and positively impacts social behaviors like relaxation, trust, and overall psychological stability.

- **Serotonin**: This hormone boosts mood and affects memory, fear, stress response, digestion, addiction, sexuality, sleep, breathing, and body temperature.

- **Endorphins**: The body's natural painkillers, released in response to pain or stress, create a feeling of well-being. They mimic the actions of opioid painkillers and are responsible for the "runner's high."

Dance has always been part of human culture, rituals, and celebrations. So why not start dancing to generate these happy hormones? With a mindset of "who cares" and stepping out of our comfort zones, we should practice dancing in an enjoyable way to stay physically active and fit.

After joining ACD, I was initially reluctant to do all the dance moves Sameer was teaching.

During an evening chit-chat with our dance coach, Tiru Sameer Yarlagadda, he revealed that he started teaching dance at just ten years old. Despite holding a B. Tech in ECE and an MBA from North Eastern Hill University, Shillong, his first love has always been dance.

Sameer's greatest breakthrough came when he learned to balance multiple responsibilities, becoming mentally and physically strong with a remarkable boost in immunity. His goal is to make the whole of India dance, with a mission to teach 75% of the Indian population.

Wow! Why not join Sameer's team like I did? You'll be amazed to discover why dance is so important for overall health.

After knowing Sameer a bit, while he showed us video clips of two ladies, aged 83 and 75, dancing to the song "Nato Nato," I was speechless!

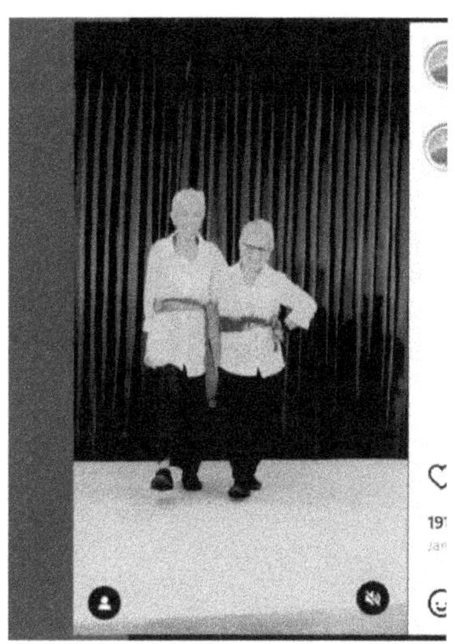

In 2003, a study in the New England Journal of Medicine found that dance can significantly improve brain health. The study, conducted by researchers at the Albert Einstein College of Medicine, investigated the effects of leisure activities on the risk of dementia in the elderly. Out of 11 types of physical activity, only dance lowered the risk of dementia. The researchers noted that dancing involves mental effort and social interaction, reducing the risk of dementia.

A 2012 study at North Dakota's Minot State University found that the Latin-style dance program Zumba improves mood and cognitive skills, such as visual recognition and decision-making. Other studies show that dance reduces stress, increases serotonin levels, and helps develop new neural connections, especially in areas involved in executive function, long-term memory, and spatial recognition.

Still not convinced? My wife used to laugh at me, saying "Xekelir mukhe xukan diya" (an Assamese proverb meaning: giving sugarcane to a person with no teeth). But here are research-backed ways dancing can improve your health:

1. **Dance Boosts Cardiovascular Health**: A 2016 study found that moderate-intensity dancing reduces the risk of heart disease by 46% compared to nondancers.

2. **Dancing Builds Core Strength**: Dance promotes good posture and prevents muscle injuries and back pain.

3. **Dance Promotes Flexibility**: Many forms of dance stretch the limbs, improving flexibility and balance.

4. **Dance Can Help With Weight Loss**: Dancing burns calories and supports weight loss. Depending on the dance style and body weight, 30 minutes of dancing can burn between 90 and 252 calories.

5. **Dancing Is Good for Bone Health**: As a weight-bearing activity, dance helps maintain bone density and can even reverse some osteoporosis damage.

6. **Dancing May Help Prevent Memory Loss**: Social dancing can reduce the risk of cognitive decline and dementia.

7. **Dance Is Good for Mental Health**: Dance can decrease anxiety, increase self-esteem, and improve psychological well-being.

8. **Dance Can Help Bust Stress**: Dancing can effectively reduce stress levels.

9. **Dance Can Help Us Feel More Socially Connected**: Dancing fosters social interaction and connectedness, crucial for mental and physical health.

So, my dear reader, when you next time hear the Gujarati song "Gotilo gotilo ... Khalasi" by Aditya Gadhvi, just hit the dance floor and let loose. If you want to maximize calorie burn, consider taking a dance cardio class. Ultimately, dancing will help you rise as a healthier person.

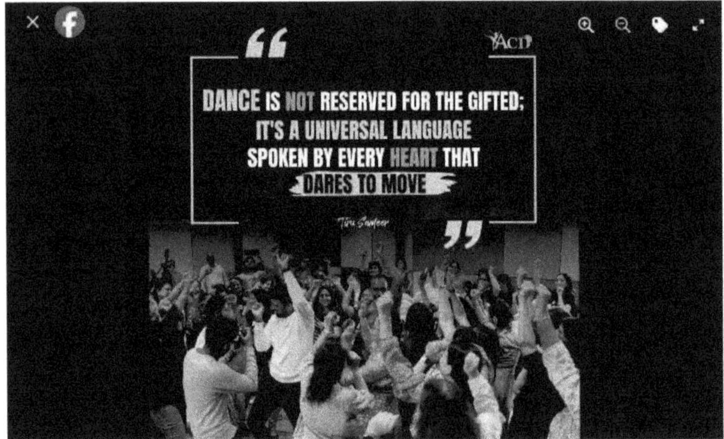

End.